MW00960497

FOOD ALLERGIES

How to Eat Well with Food Allergies: A Comprehensive Guide to Diagnosis, Treatment, and Beyond

JACE COOPER

Copyright © 2024 By Jace Cooper

All Rights Reserved.

Table of Contents

Introductory

An abnormal immune reaction to a specific food or substance in food is what is known as a food allergy. Food allergies occur when an individual's immune system incorrectly interprets particular proteins in the allergenic food as harmful intruders, either through ingestion or contact. In response, the immune system releases molecules like histamine, which can set off a cascade of unpleasant effects, including but not limited to allergies.

Depending on the severity of the allergy, the following are some of the most common symptoms:

1. Skin reactions: Hives, itching, or eczema.

- Nausea, vomiting, diarrhea, or stomach discomforts are all examples of gastrointestinal symptoms.

Sneezing, coughing, wheezing, difficulty breathing and a runny or stuffy nose are all examples of respiratory symptoms.

- **Anaphylaxis:** a severe and sometimes fatal allergic reaction characterized by a sudden and dramatic drop in blood pressure, swelling of the throat, and trouble breathing.

• Some people with food allergies only need a very small amount of the allergenic item to experience symptoms, but this is not the case for everyone. Peanuts, tree nuts, eggs, milk, wheat, soy, fish, and shellfish are only some of the most commonly reported food allergies. Individuals with the same food allergy may experience different types and degrees of reaction.

Those who suffer from food allergies must steer clear of the offending substances and have emergency treatment on hand, such as epinephrine (available as EpiPen) in case of an anaphylactic reaction. Maintaining one's health and safety often necessitates the assistance of an allergist or immunologist in the identification and treatment of food allergies.

CHAPTER ONE
Allergens in the Food Supply

Specific foods or food ingredients often cause allergy reactions in susceptible people are known as common food allergens. Most cases of food allergy can be traced back to these substances. Some of the most prevalent allergens in the food supply are as follows:

• One of the most common and life-threatening food allergies is to peanuts. For those who are allergic, even a trace of peanut might be fatal.

• Almonds, walnuts, cashews, and pistachios are all examples of tree nuts. These nuts can cause serious allergies that often last a lifetime.

• Most youngsters outgrow milk allergies as they get older. Proteins in cow's milk, such as casein and whey, can trigger an allergic reaction in certain people.

• Eggs are a common allergen in children, and the reactions to them can range from minor hives to life-threatening anaphylaxis. Typically, it's the egg whites that cause reactions.

• Allergies to wheat can cause anything from rashes and stomach pain to life-threatening anaphylaxis.

They differ from celiac disease intolerance to gluten) in significant ways.

• Allergies to soybeans are common in children and can manifest in a number of ways. It can be difficult to avoid soy because it is used in so many processed goods.

• **Fish:** many people have allergies to seafood like salmon, tuna, and cod. Fish allergens are prevalent in many unexpected foods and can cause severe reactions.

Allergies to shellfish fall into two categories: Mollusks and crustaceans such as shrimp, crab, and lobster. Both are potential allergens.

The intensity of allergy reactions varies widely from person to person, and some people are sensitive to many dietary allergens. Avoidance of allergenic foods and other forms of management are essential for those who suffer from food allergies. An allergist or immunologist should be seen if you think you have a food allergy so that you can get a proper diagnosis and individualized treatment plan.

Food Allergy Diagnosis

A healthcare provider, often an allergist or immunologist, will use a combination of the patient's medical history, a physical examination, and specialized testing to diagnose food allergies. Common procedures for identifying food allergies include the following:

• A thorough medical history is typically the first step. The patient gives a detailed account of their symptoms, including when they manifest, how long they last, and the foods they believe are to blame. It may be helpful to know whether there is an allergy history in your family.

• The second step is a physical exam, where the doctor will search for symptoms of allergies including hives, dermatitis, or breathing problems.

• Third, an elimination diet may be employed in some situations. Eliminating potentially problematic foods from the diet for a set amount of time, and then slowly reintroducing them to check for a return of symptoms. A medical expert's supervision is required for this procedure.

Allergen extract (such as a diluted food protein) is applied to the skin (often the forearm or back) in a skin prick test. After that, a tiny needle is used to pierce the skin and inject the allergen just under the surface. Within 15–20 minutes of testing, the patient may develop a small, raised bump or hives if they are allergic to the chemical.

• **Blood Tests:** Blood tests, such as the specific IgE (immunoglobulin E) test, can assess the levels of IgE antibodies to specific dietary allergens. Indicators of food allergy include elevated IgE levels.

The oral food challenge is the most accurate way to identify food allergies. Under medical supervision, the person consumes small amounts of the potentially allergic food. When previous tests have failed to provide a definitive diagnosis, this one is a must.

Patch testing is used for the diagnosis of contact dermatitis, which occurs when an allergen comes into direct contact with the skin. Food allergy testing does not commonly use this method.

- **Component-Resolved Diagnostics:** IgE antibodies to specific components of allergenic foods can be identified using specific IgE testing in some situations. This can assist differentiate between cross-reactive allergens and genuine allergies.

Some tests for food allergies may provide false positives or false negatives due to the difficulty of making the diagnosis. Thus, it is recommended that an allergist assess the results and make a final diagnosis. Accurate testing and individualized counsel on managing food allergies, including dietary restrictions and the use of epinephrine in the event of a severe reaction, can only be obtained by seeing an allergist or immunologist.

Food Allergy Management

Multiple approaches are used to manage food allergies, all with the goal of protecting those who suffer from them from dangerous reactions. Managing food allergies requires taking the following measures:

• The first and foremost action is to get a proper diagnosis from a medical expert, usually an allergist or immunologist. This will aid in determining the nature and extent of the individual's food allergy.

• Second, the key tactic is to refrain from eating the offending items altogether. This necessitates paying close attention to food labels, inquiring about restaurant menu items' components, and avoiding potential sources of cross-contamination.

• **Education:** Individuals with food allergies, as well as their caregivers, should be informed on the individual allergens and how to spot probable sources of allergens in food products.

For those with life-threatening food allergies, a doctor may recommend carrying an epinephrine autoinjector (such an EpiPen) at all times. In the event of an anaphylactic reaction, these tools can be crucial. Get familiar with them and always have them on hand.

• Create and stick to a tailored allergy action plan that details what to do in the event of an allergic reaction. Tell your loved ones and your caretakers about this strategy.

• Medical Alert Jewelry: In the event of an emergency, it is a good idea to wear a bracelet or necklace that indicates the wearer has a food allergy.

• Safe Food Preparation: If you have a food-allergic child, consider creating a dedicated room for food preparation and using separate utensils and equipment to prevent cross-contamination.

• Communicate your food sensitivities to the wait staff or hosts at restaurants and social occasions. Inquire about the food's ingredients and how it was prepared to avoid getting sick.

• Replace allergenic foods in your diet with safer options, as discussed in point #9. You can find many of allergy-friendly products in stores, and cooking at home is easy when you avoid common allergens.

• Ongoing Monitoring: The best way to keep track of your condition, address any changes in your allergies, and revise your action plan is to schedule regular follow-up sessions with your allergist.

Join a local or virtual community for people with food allergies. The knowledge, comfort, and camaraderie gained from these sources are invaluable.

Know the regulations in your nation about food labeling. Common allergens are required to be listed prominently on food labels in some areas, making it simpler to find suitable options.

Travelers with food allergies should plan ahead by learning about allergen-free restaurants and emergency medical facilities.

Keep in mind that some people with food allergies have more severe reactions than others. You must take them seriously, always be on the lookout, and have a plan in place in case of an allergic reaction. For optimal management of food allergies, it is essential to consult with medical experts.

CHAPTER TWO
Allergy Suffering as a Way of Life

Living with food allergies can bring unique obstacles, but with proper management and safeguards, persons with food allergies can have healthy and fulfilling lives. Here are some strategies for coping with food allergies in everyday life:

- **Academics:** Acquiring information is crucial. Find out what foods you can and can't eat, what allergenic components to avoid, and what rules and regulations govern food labeling.

- always read the labels on processed and packaged goods. You can find potential allergy sources by reading the warning labels and ingredient lists. Keep in mind that allergic substances might go by a variety of names.

- if you or a member of your home suffers from food allergies, you should take extra precautions when preparing meals. Keep raw and cooked foods separate by using individual cutting boards, utensils, and pots and pans.

Communicate your food sensitivities to the wait staff or host at any social occasions you attend.

Feel free to inquire about the origins of any ingredients or processes used in the production of your meal.

• Always have recommended emergency drugs (such as epinephrine auto-injectors) available. Make sure you and your loved ones are familiar with their proper use in the event of an allergic reaction.

• Make and stick to an allergy action plan that you and your loved ones (including teachers, aides, and classmates) come up with together. In the event of an allergic response, the actions outlined here will come in handy.

• In case of an emergency where you are unable to speak, medical staff and first responders will know about your food allergies if you wear medical alert jewelry.

• Allergen-Free Snacks Always have some safe snacks on hand, in case you find yourself in a scenario where you won't have access to your regular diet.

• Look into substitutes and recipes for foods that don't include your allergens. There are a lot of options for those with food allergies, including products and recipes.

• assemble a backup plan by joining local and online food allergy support groups. These groups can be a great resource for learning new things, getting emotional support, and making new friends.

• Stay away from potentially hazardous situations: use extra caution in settings where cross-contamination is likely, such as potlucks, communal kitchens, and buffets.

• If your child has food allergies, it is important to teach them how to self-manage their condition, identify allergic foods, and express their requirements at an age-appropriate level.

• **Be a Wise Traveler:** Prepare thoroughly before leaving on a trip. Find out what options there are for those with food allergies at your location, and pack a small first aid kit in case of an emergency.

Check in with your allergist on a frequent basis to address any changes in your allergy symptoms and to revise your allergy management plan.

Be your own best defender; number fifteen on the list. Spread information, raise awareness, and push for accommodations for those who suffer from food allergies.

The challenges of dealing with food allergies can be mitigated with awareness, planning, and support. Always keep in mind that allergies are dynamic conditions, and that you must take measures to ensure your own safety and well-being.

Conclusion

food allergies are immune system reactions to specific proteins in food, and they can cause a wide variety of symptoms, from minor discomfort to severe and life-threatening reactions. Allergic reactions are common among those who eat foods containing peanuts, tree nuts, milk, eggs, wheat, soy, fish, or shellfish.

• Skin prick tests, blood testing, and oral food challenges are just a few of the diagnostic tools available for identifying food allergies. The severity and specific dietary allergy require a precise diagnosis.

Avoiding foods known to trigger reactions is the first and most important step in managing food allergies. Be ready for possible allergic responses by always having emergency medication on hand, such as epinephrine.

Life with food allergies takes ongoing monitoring, but with the correct knowledge, support, and safeguards, it is possible to live a healthy and fulfilling life. The best way to deal with food allergies and make sure you're safe is to educate yourself, tell people about your condition, and take preventative measures.

THE END